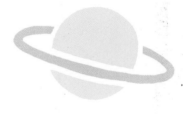

this is the story of

_____

my parent(s)

Their name(s) _____

_____

PHOTOS & MEMENTOS

A few things to know about them _____

_____

_____

_____

PHOTOS & MEMENTOS

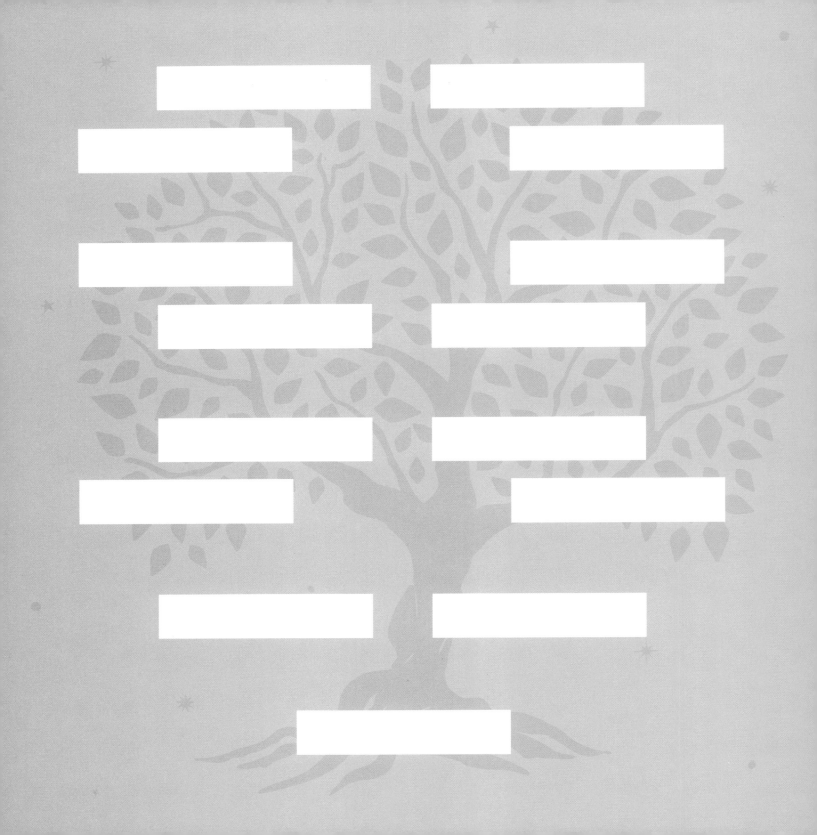

my family

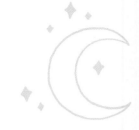

Some things to know about my family _____

_____

_____

_____

PHOTOS & MEMENTOS

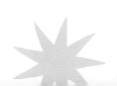

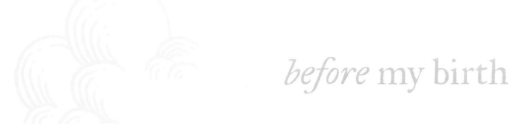

before my birth

How my family prepared for me _____

_____

_____

_____

PHOTOS & MEMENTOS

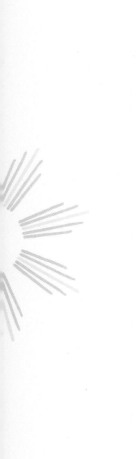

PHOTOS & MEMENTOS

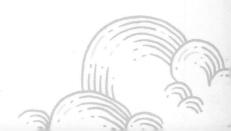

MY HANDPRINT(S)
AND/OR FOOTPRINT(S)

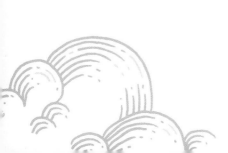

all about my arrival

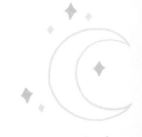

My name _____

Its meaning _____

My birthplace _____

Birthdate _____ Time _____

Length _____ Weight _____

Memories of our first moments together _____

_____

_____

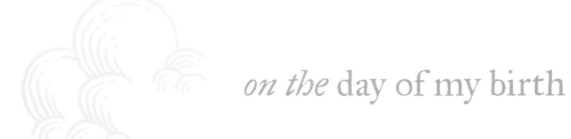

on the day of my birth

The most popular song _____

Our nation's leader _____

The cost of a cup of coffee _____

The top news headlines _____

_____

Other special things about this day _____

_____

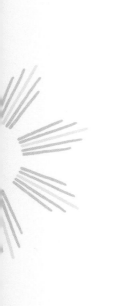

PHOTOS & MEMENTOS

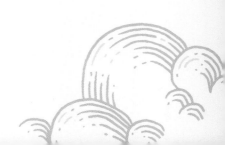

monthly
MILESTONES

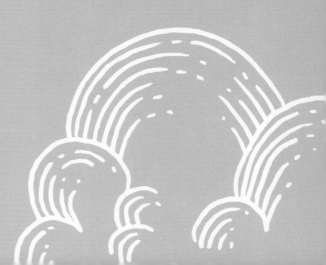

month one

I love _____

_____

_____

_____

I don't like _____

_____

_____

_____

I learned _____

_____

_____

_____

An unforgettable memory _____

_____

_____

_____

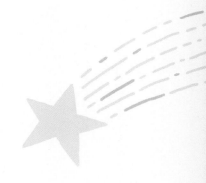

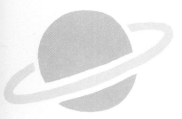

PHOTOS & MEMENTOS

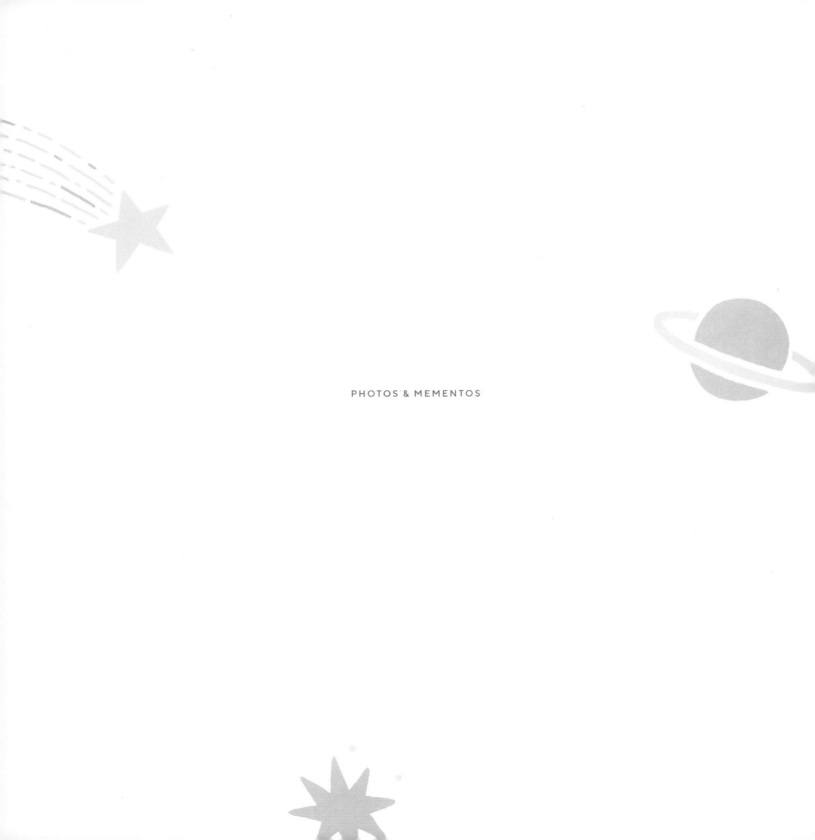

PHOTOS & MEMENTOS

month two

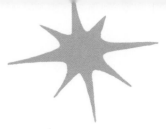

I love _____

_____

_____

_____

I don't like _____

_____

_____

_____

I learned _____

_____

_____

_____

An unforgettable memory _____

_____

_____

_____

month three

I love _____

_____

_____

_____

I don't like _____

_____

_____

_____

I learned _____

_____

_____

_____

An unforgettable memory _____

_____

_____

_____

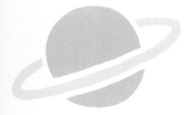

PHOTOS & MEMENTOS

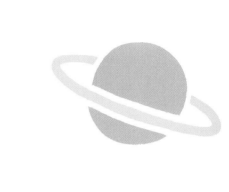

PHOTOS & MEMENTOS

month four

I love _____

_____

_____

_____

I don't like _____

_____

_____

_____

I learned _____

_____

_____

_____

An unforgettable memory _____

_____

_____

_____

month five

I love _____

_____

_____

_____

I don't like _____

_____

_____

_____

I learned _____

_____

_____

_____

An unforgettable memory _____

_____

_____

_____

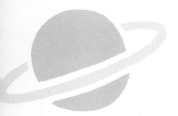

PHOTOS & MEMENTOS

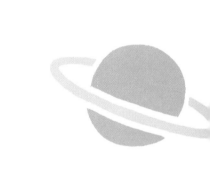

PHOTOS & MEMENTOS

month six

I love _____

_____

_____

_____

I don't like _____

_____

_____

_____

I learned _____

_____

_____

_____

An unforgettable memory _____

_____

_____

_____

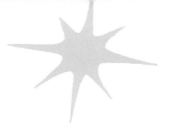

month seven

I love _____

_____

_____

_____

I don't like _____

_____

_____

_____

I learned _____

_____

_____

_____

An unforgettable memory _____

_____

_____

_____

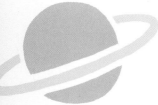

PHOTOS & MEMENTOS

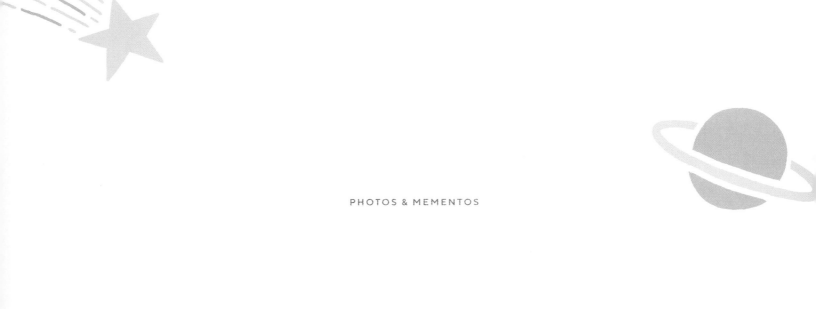

PHOTOS & MEMENTOS

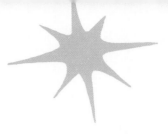

month eight

I love _____

_____

_____

_____

I don't like _____

_____

_____

_____

I learned _____

_____

_____

_____

An unforgettable memory _____

_____

_____

_____

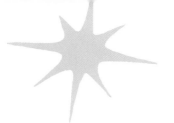

month nine

I love _____

_____

_____

_____

I don't like _____

_____

_____

_____

I learned _____

_____

_____

_____

An unforgettable memory _____

_____

_____

_____

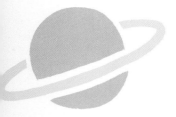

PHOTOS & MEMENTOS

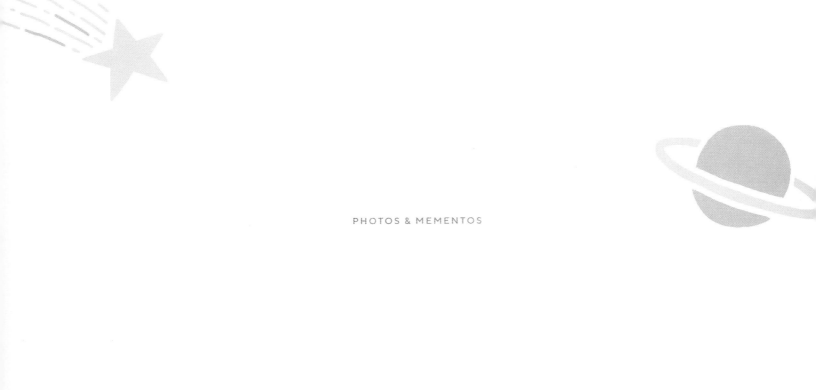

PHOTOS & MEMENTOS

month ten

I love _____

_____

_____

_____

I don't like _____

_____

_____

_____

I learned _____

_____

_____

_____

An unforgettable memory _____

_____

_____

_____

month eleven

I love _____

_____

_____

_____

I don't like _____

_____

_____

_____

I learned _____

_____

_____

_____

An unforgettable memory _____

_____

_____

_____

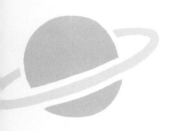

PHOTOS & MEMENTOS

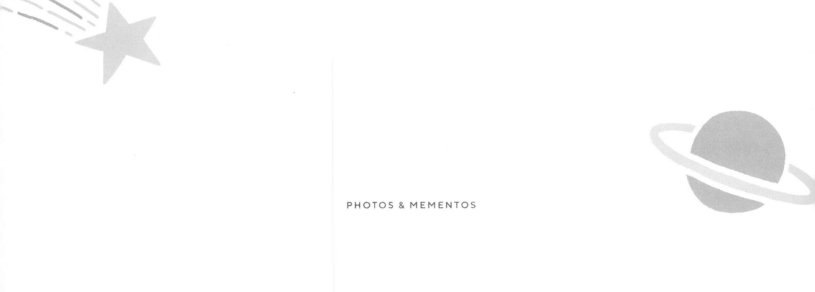

PHOTOS & MEMENTOS

month twelve

I love _____

_____

_____

_____

I don't like _____

_____

_____

_____

I learned _____

_____

_____

_____

An unforgettable memory _____

_____

_____

_____

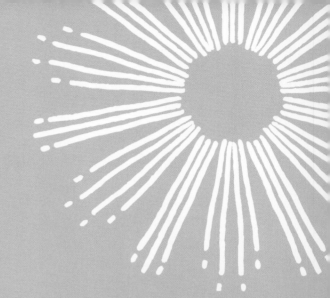

meaningful
FIRSTS

my first bath

PHOTOS & MEMENTOS

my first outing

PHOTOS & MEMENTOS

my first smile

PHOTOS & MEMENTOS

my first laugh

PHOTOS & MEMENTOS

my first tooth

PHOTOS & MEMENTOS

my first solid food

PHOTOS & MEMENTOS

my first time sitting up

PHOTOS & MEMENTOS

my first time crawling

PHOTOS & MEMENTOS

my first time standing

PHOTOS & MEMENTOS

my first steps

_____

PHOTOS & MEMENTOS

my first word

PHOTOS & MEMENTOS

my first haircut

PHOTOS & MEMENTOS

my first
_____

_____

PHOTOS & MEMENTOS

my first

_____

_____

PHOTOS & MEMENTOS

holidays and
CELEBRATIONS

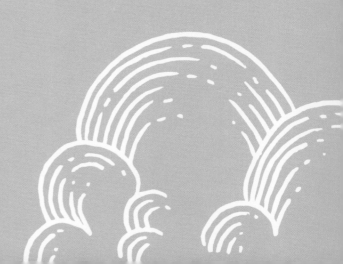

my first

SUGGESTION:

new year's

PHOTOS & MEMENTOS

my first

_____

SUGGESTION:

valentine's day

PHOTOS & MEMENTOS

my first

_____

SUGGESTION:

st. patrick's day

PHOTOS & MEMENTOS

my first

_____

SUGGESTION:

independence day

PHOTOS & MEMENTOS

my first
_____

SUGGESTION:

mother's day

PHOTOS & MEMENTOS

my first

SUGGESTION:

father's day

PHOTOS & MEMENTOS

my first

_____

SUGGESTION:

halloween

PHOTOS & MEMENTOS

my first

_____

SUGGESTION:

thanksgiving

PHOTOS & MEMENTOS

my first

_____

PHOTOS & MEMENTOS

my first

_____

PHOTOS & MEMENTOS

my first

_____

PHOTOS & MEMENTOS

my first

_____

PHOTOS & MEMENTOS

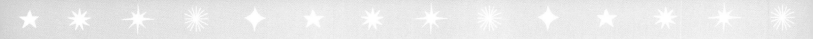

my first birthday

PHOTOS & MEMENTOS

How we celebrated _____

_____

_____

People who celebrated with me _____

_____

a few of my favorite things

Song _____   Book _____

Food _____   Toy _____

Activities _____

_____

PHOTOS & MEMENTOS

PHOTOS & MEMENTOS

PHOTOS & MEMENTOS

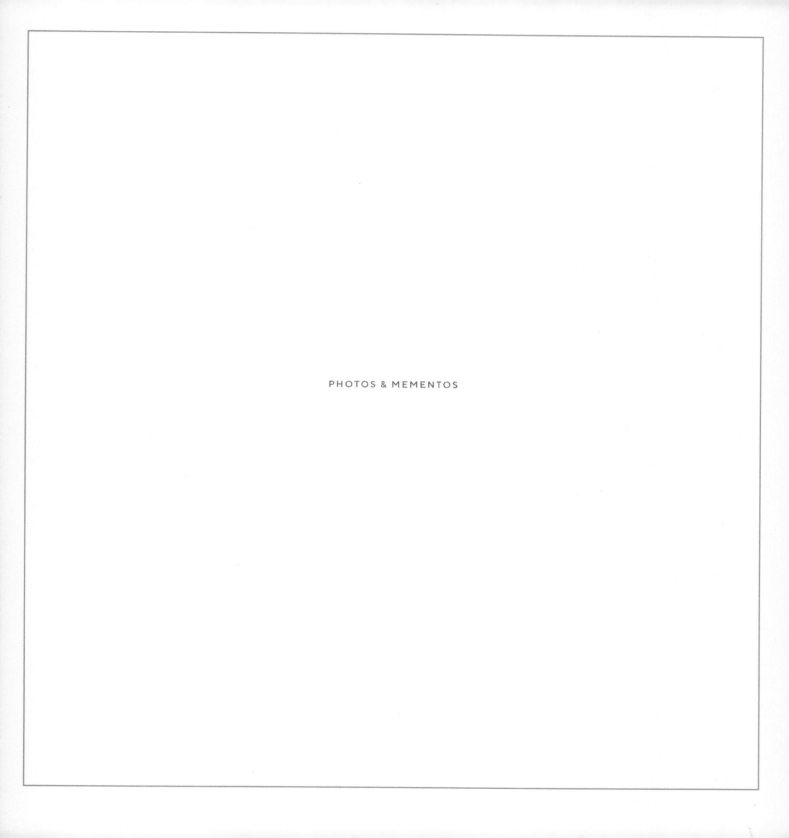

PHOTOS & MEMENTOS

Zeitgeist™ is a trademark of Penguin Random House LLC
ISBN: 9780593690284

Art by Rough Edges Supply/CreativeMarket.com
and ekosuwandono/Shutterstock.com
Book design by Lauren Smith
Edited by Clara Song Lee

Manufactured in China
1st Printing